YOUR KNOWLEDGE HAS VALUE

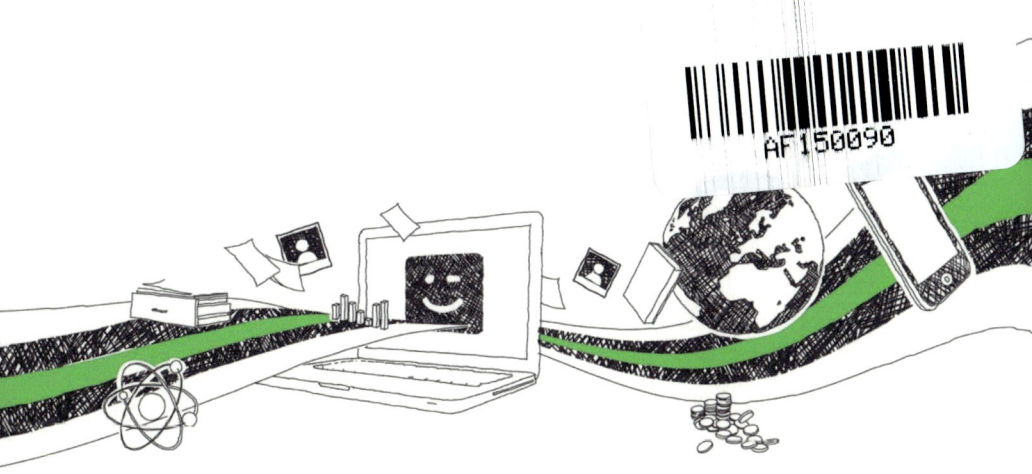

- We will publish your bachelor's and master's thesis, essays and papers

- Your own eBook and book - sold worldwide in all relevant shops

- Earn money with each sale

Upload your text at www.GRIN.com and publish for free

Mohamed Sood

Is there any connection between poverty and the prevalence of HIV and AIDS?

GRIN Verlag

Bibliografische Information der Deutschen Nationalbibliothek:

Die Deutsche Bibliothek verzeichnet diese Publikation in der Deutschen National-
bibliografie; detaillierte bibliografische Daten sind im Internet über http://dnb.d-
nb.de/ abrufbar.

Imprint:

Copyright © 2013 GRIN Verlag GmbH
Druck und Bindung: Books on Demand GmbH, Norderstedt Germany
ISBN: 978-3-656-48202-4

This book at GRIN:

http://www.grin.com/en/e-book/215379/is-there-any-connection-between-poverty-
and-the-prevalence-of-hiv-and-aids

GRIN - Your knowledge has value

Der GRIN Verlag publiziert seit 1998 wissenschaftliche Arbeiten von Studenten, Hochschullehrern und anderen Akademikern als eBook und gedrucktes Buch. Die Verlagswebsite www.grin.com ist die ideale Plattform zur Veröffentlichung von Hausarbeiten, Abschlussarbeiten, wissenschaftlichen Aufsätzen, Dissertationen und Fachbüchern.

Visit us on the internet:

http://www.grin.com/

http://www.facebook.com/grincom

http://www.twitter.com/grin_com

Is there any connection between poverty and the prevalence of HIV and AIDS?

The connection between poverty and HIV and it's a marriage that needs to be prevented.

To understand the relationship one has to make sense of the complex socio-economic processes in the society and not forgetting conceptualization of poverty which is multi-dimensional. Poverty actually completes the vicious cycle of HIV.

The estimated number of people living with HIV in 2009 was estimated to be around 33.3 million by the United Nation Program on HIV/AIDS(UNAIDS), in sub-Saharan Africa two thirds are infected with HIV and they are from lower socio-economical groups, with women affected more than men(Regional Statistic for HIV and AIDS, 2009)

 High percentage of population living on less than 1 dollar per day have a higher HIV prevalence as shown by the data provided by UNAIDS. (Global Report, 2006) Industrialized countries have lower HIV prevalence, compared to countries with high percentage of population living below 1 dollar. The graph below shows the relationship between poverty and HIV.

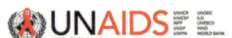

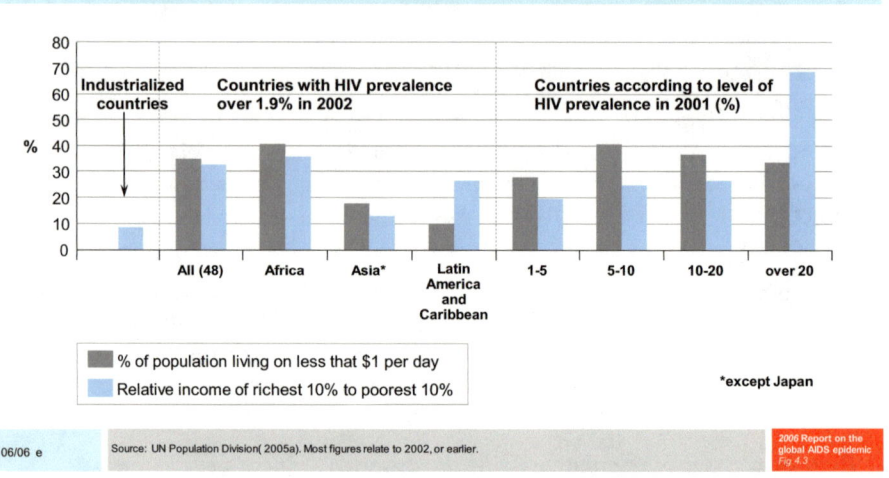

Sub-Saharan Africa is the world poorest region and it accounts for more than 60 percent of people living with HIV. People living with HIV in Sub-Sahara Africa are poor reflects that the epidemic has now spread. (Piot p, Greener R, Russell S, 2007) More than 14000 people are daily infected with HIV and 11000 are dying due to HIV/AIDS related illness in sub-Saharan Africa (World Health Organization, 2005)

Access to HIV treatment and prevention services is a challenge among poor and marginalized populations living with HIV. People infected with HIV, who receive treatment, survive on average 27.8 years instead of 11.7 years expected in the absence of treatment (United Nation Population Division, 2008 Revision).

Poverty plays a role in the transmission in HIV. First, poor people are more susceptible to HIV due to malnutrition that leads to weakened immune system and increase the chance of sexual transmitted infections and general poor health. The risk of infection with HIV heightened by high prevalence of such cofactors like nutrition, stress, which decrease immune response in HIV- negative persons and increase viral load in HIV- infected persons (Stillwaggon, 2006)

In United States, a report based on interviews of more than 9,000 people conducted in poor areas 23 U.S cities among heterosexuals, found that 2.1 percent of them had HIV. The findings showed strong evidence of a link between poverty and HIV infection. The lack of access to medical care in low-income communities means increase in spread of the disease, people are unaware they are infected and therefore not being treated. (Roy Wilson and Betsy McKay, 2010)

Secondly, access to health care and social services is very difficult or limited because of poor infrastructure or inadequate medical supply in the regions. The poor are less likely to have knowledge of condom use, HIV testing and more likely to have untreated cofactor sexual transmitted infections.

The poorer a person is the less good his state of healthcare is likely to be. This is because poorer people are less likely to be informed about healthcare. They are less likely to have healthcare insurance and have shorter life expectancy. Daily search for survival makes them take unnecessary health risks. (HIV and AIDS Prevention, 2004)

Poverty leads to social and political exclusion. HIV programs are neglected and are of no interest to a hungry nation or individual that is rarely if ever related to their needs. It is the absence of sustainable livelihood which limits the possibilities of changing the socio-economic conditions of the poor. Unless the reality of lives of the poor are changed they will persist with behaviors which expose them to HIV infection.

Poverty decreases choices. Individuals and communities who are infected with HIV have choices to change their life style. This is circumstantial access of adequate cash and utilizes information to maintain a healthier life and productive life, compared to individuals who are financially constrained, they will have limited access to medical care when they are sick and this can lead to different modes of attaining money e.g. prostitution

Poverty causes reduced capacity to deal with mortality and morbidity. This includes the absence of savings which can help in times of death or illness. The poor are unable to meet the cost of treatment of opportunistic infections, transport cost to health care when they are ill. This either leads to them selling their possessed assets or engages in inappropriate sexual behaviors to get money.

In poor communities, sex workers are extremely vulnerable to lack of care when they are sick, as illustrated in the following quote from one of the urban sex worker: "We have no support or visits from neighbors because they regard us as outcast or no human beings because of our business.

They always wish us to die. It's not our wish to be sex workers, but it's due to poverty." (Bond et al, 2003)

 A study done by Booysen (2004), found a small percentage of women less than 4 percent, who were knowledgeable about HIV/AIDS and had engaged in risky sexual behavior. The likelihood of engaging in risky sexual behavior was higher among women from poorer households relative to those from ones that are more affluent. The majority (92%) of women stated lack of control over decision pertaining to financial issues as one of the reasons for engaging in risky sexual behavior (LS Tladi, 2006)

Susceptibility to HIV in women is further enhanced in marginalized or migrant population. The National data from Nigeria shows that the rate of infection in sex workers was 30-37 percent, compared to 4 percent in general population. In Viet Nam, Migrant workers were twice more likely to be infected and become HIV positive than other women. (Asian Development Bank, 2005)

The Vicious Cycle

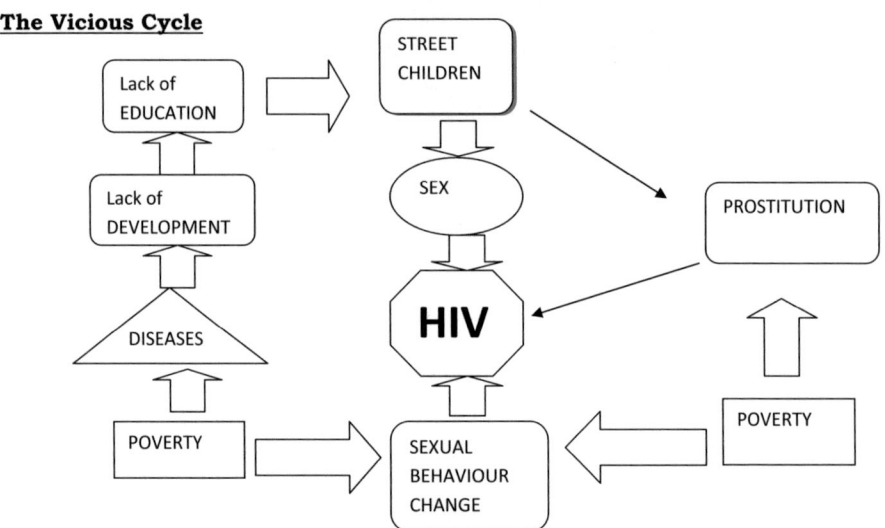

Source: Writers own

Lower social status, lower level of education, cultural and social practices are some of the factors which increase the chances of women to contract diseases and/or increases the susceptibility to HIV. Poverty is linked to sexual behavior in a number of pathways. These include transition from commercial sex, to gain of job through sexual favors, that's not even the climax. During food shortages, women may seek income through sex to actually bridge the income gap for survival and such behavior puts them at a higher risk of contracting HIV. The effects of these accounts for the much higher infection rates in young women who are increasingly unable to sustain themselves by other work in either the formal or the informal sectors.

Physical dislocation of families, driven by the need to find work, coupled with the ability to move around via relatively good transport routes, probably play a large part in transmission of HIV. Men tend to live away from home for long periods, increasing the chances of both partners engaging in commercial sex. Strong urban– rural economic linkages in southern Africa may translate in to both higher income and high rate of infection. The links between livelihood and risk suggest that HIV is an 'occupational hazard' for particular economic categories of people (Bryceson and Fonseca, Stuart Gillespie, 2005)

Worldwide women account for half of the people living with HIV. Sixty percent of women living with HIV are found in sub-Sahara Africa, and three out of four of the infected are young females under the age of 25 years. (UNFPA, 2009)

Children take responsibilities of an adult, because the parents are either sick or deceased. The survival depends on either engaging in sexual favors to earn income. One fundamental difficulty with teenage marriages due to poverty makes the girl dependant on their husbands and therefore, they lack the power to make demands from them. They cannot ask their husbands to get an HIV test; they cannot abstain from intercourse or demand condom use; they cannot insist that their husband be monogamous; and ultimately; they cannot leave because they cannot repay their dowry. In addition, returning to their parents' home may not be an option because divorce has never been considered culturally acceptable and leaving their husbands may have serious implications on the social or tribal ties that were developed during the marriage.

HIV prevalence in Moshi Tanzania was high among young women who started having sex at early ages, less than 15 years old. The prevalence peaked early at 10 percent among 25-29 year old. This suggests that most infections in women occur at a younger age, during the first few years after sexual encounter. Immature genital tract and cervical ectopy, which is common in young women, might increase the risk. Untreated sexually transmitted disease may increase the biological susceptibility. Young women mostly have older partners who may likely be previously infected. Therefore, poverty remains the root of early marriages for most young girls in Africa (UNAIDS, 2004)

Countries in civil wars like Sudan show symptoms of child related social stress, increase in child slavery and trafficking, increase in numbers on street children, very young prostitutes, child neglect and abandonment which can lead to increase level of HIV infections (UNICEF, 2001)

HIV infection and poverty deeply intertwine. As the burden of caring for the sick, the dying and the orphaned forces millions of African women deeper into poverty and batters their energy and self-esteem, so it increases the pressure to resort to high risk 'transactional sex'. Sex in exchange for money, goods and sex with 'older sugar daddies', offer the illusion of material security as more and more women and girls take to streets as their only means of survival. [The UN secretary General Task force On HIV/AIDS in Southern Africa UNAIDS, Geneva, 2008) Individuals and extended families have largely met the caretaking burden of HIV in developing countries.

The number of children infected with HIV is high due to perinatal transmission. This is easily preventable through appropriate access to drugs Highly Active Antiretroviral Therapy (HAART); these drugs are not accessible due to poor infrastructure in the rural areas and the consequence of this is the high transmission rate of HIV.

Breast feeding, accounts for significant number of babies, been infected with HIV. This is avoidable but poverty is clearly a major hurdle in prevention of the transmission to the babies. To prevent the transmission alternative mode of feeding is recommended but this requires the ability to buy the formula milk, access clean water, access fuel for preparation of the formula and above all empowerment through education to understand why these changes have to be made from breast feeding to formula milk. It's clear that breast milk is readily available, ready to drink, no need of fuel to make it warm. Neither clean water nor income is available to buy formula milk in poor setting and the next best option is too continue breast feeding which increases the rate of transmission. All this happens because of poverty.

The shift of rural to urban migration in search of better payments leads to mobile population which often consist of the large numbers of young men and women who often don't find the jobs they are looking for and therefore engage in risky behavior with obvious consequences in terms of HIV.

The lack of economic opportunities in many of Africa's rural areas has long induced men (and increasingly women) to migrate to urban and other wages centre in search of work, especially in southern Africa where seasonal or temporary migration brings migrants home to their families regularly, probably facilitating the rapid spread of HIV. In South Africa, for example, HIV prevalence was twice as high among migrant's workers (26%) compared to nonimmigrant workers (Crush 2001; Lurie, et al, 2003). Large –scale migration in the context of impoverishment, deep socioeconomic inequalities and social dislocation appears to be an ideal for the spread of HIV/AIDS and other sexually transmitted infections (Kark 1949; Myer, Morroni and Susser, 2003). Very high infection levels have been reported in areas beside major transport routes, at border crossings, near military bases and around mines and agricultural estates (International organization For Migration, 2003)

Low socio-economic status robs the poor of the knowledge necessary to prevent transmission of infection by practicing safer sexual behavior. This has affected many countries, communities; by loosing large number of labourers, teachers and working force of the nation, leading to catastrophic effects for health and educational systems and every economic sector in the country.

In Botswana, the economic growth is projected to decline from 1.2 percent to 2.0 percent over a period 2001-2021 due to HIV/AIDS. This will result in fall in economy from 23 to 35 percent smaller than expected. (UNDP, 2007)

Prevention and treatment can help people with HIV infection to maintain or reassume productive economic activity. Tea pickers who were HIV infected in Kenya showed rapid improvement in labour productivity after starting antiretroviral treatment for 12 months. (UNFPA, 2009)

Conclusion

The HIV epidemic has its deep roots in poverty, unless poverty is eradicated or reduced, there will be little progress in the fight against HIV transmission and the consequences of unstable economy.

Poverty eradication and employment programs should be directly linked to sexual reproductive health and HIV programs

Empower people with knowledge on HIV and strategies on income generation programs, which can help them, sustain life and support the families.

HIV related needs of migrants should be addressed, refugees and displaced persons during civil wars.

Community networks like community based organizations; religious groups should be supported in empowering the community.

Invest in increased access to affordable medical care for all people and supportive services. Medical personal should be trained to improve awareness on HIV/AIDS on women.

Reference:

1. Worldwide HIV & AIDS statistics: www. Avert.org/worlstats.htm
2. UNAIDS;
   http://www.data.unaids.org/pub/GlobalReport/2006globalreportslide029.ppt
3. Peter Piot, Robert greener, Sarah Russell, squaring the circle: Aids, Poverty, And Human development in PLoS medicine
   http://medicine.plosjournals.org/perlserv/?request=get-document&doi=10.1371/journal.pmed.00403147cr=1#journal-pmed-0040314-b004
4. WHO annual report Global HIV/AIDS overview Geneva(Switzerland):WHO;2005
5. United Nation Population Division, 2008 Revision
6. Aids and the Ecology of Poverty by Eileen Stillwaggon 2006 p.31
7. The Wall Street Journal,
   http://online.wsj.com/article/SB10001424052748704875004575375070903484974.html
8. HIV and AIDS Prevention by Dr Prince Efere 2nd Edition 2004 p.16
9. Stigma When There Is No Other Option: Understanding How poverty Fuels Discrimination towards People Living with HIV in Zambia by Virginia Bond p.188
10. Poverty and HIV/AIDS in South Africa: an empirical contribution
    www.sahara.org.za/download/250-poverty-poverty-hivaids-in-south-africa-an-empirical-contribution.html
11. Asian Development Bank (2005) Gender Network News. Special issue: Perspective on gender and HIV/AIDS.
    http://www.adb.org/documents/periodicals/GNN/newsletter-13.pdf.
12. AIDS, Poverty, and Hunger: Challenges and Responses by Stuart Gillespie 2005 p.23
13. UNFPA 2009,
    http://www.unfpa.org/public/cache/offonce/factsheet/pid/3849#fn11
14. USAID annual report available:
    http://www.usaid.gov/our_work/humanitarian_assistance/disaster_assistance/publications/annual_reports/index.html
15. United Nation Programme on HIV and AIDS; World AIDS Campaign 2004; women, girls, HIV and AIDS. http://data.unaids.org/WAC/wac-2004_stategynote_en.pdf
16. WHO HIV/AIDS global review Geneva(Switzerland);WHO; 2006
17. Economical Factors; http://www.icaso.org/publications/gender_EN_4.pdf

18. Joint United Nations Programme on HIV/AIDS, 2008 Report on the Global Aids Epidemic, UNAIDS, Geneva, 2008
19. UNDP, The Economic Impact of HIV/AIDS in Botswana, March 2007. http://www.unbotswana.org.bw/undp/docs/economic_impact_study_execec utive_summaryfinal.
20. Poverty and HIV/AIDS in sub-Saharan Africa, Desmond Cohen. http://library.unesco-iicba.org/English/HIV_AIDS/cdrom%20materials/poverty.htm
21. UNAIDS. What Countries Need: Investments needed for 2010 targets. http://data.unaids.org/pub/report/2009/20090210_investments_needed_2 010_en.pdf